Reflexology

The Absolute Beginners Manual that Will Help Weight Loss, Eliminate Tension, and Relieve Pain by Applying Reflexology Techniques from Ancient Times

By

Isaiah Seber

© 2016

Table of Contents

Introduction: Reflexology – Nature's Ancient Cure

Have you been suffering from aches and pains? Are you suffering from an illness or injury? Are you having a hard time losing weight or controlling your anxiety? If you've answered 'yes' to at least one of these questions, you might want to know a little secret. It may just be the most impactful secret you'll hear your entire life, so listen carefully. Those medications that you may be taking (or considering taking) for your aches and pains, injuries, illness, weight loss, or anxiety may not be exactly what you need to achieve your goal of healing your body or feeling better.

Traditional medicine has come a long way in the last few decades, but that does not mean that the practice is perfect. What if you found out that there are some much more powerful treatment methods that can help cure you and can benefit your body and mind in many additional ways?

The Healing Power of Nature

Nature actually holds some of the most powerful cures for a myriad of illnesses, diseases, injuries, and other ailments. The pharmaceutical industry, for the most part, has been working hard for a very long time to keep this simple little fact a secret so that they can make more money off of the chemical concoctions they create. But, they couldn't keep the secret forever. More and more people today are understanding the healing power of nature and turning to ancient, natural techniques to recover from injuries, diseases, and psychological troubles, as well as assist them with losing weight in the healthiest ways.

This brings us to reflexology. You've probably heard the term in passing at some point throughout your life, but what exactly is it? Let's take a closer look.

Reflexology – Heal Your Body with Your Body

Wait, what? Yes, you read that right. Our bodies are amazing. Every little part of our bodies are connected with a lot of other parts that all work and function together to help us live, heal, and grow throughout every moment of every day without us even noticing. When you consider the unbelievable feats our bodies perform naturally (just think about what our digestive system does for us, or our skin – the largest organ of the body), it's easy to understand that there are certain ways for us to manipulate our bodies to promote healing – we just need to know what those techniques are and how to use them.

Reflexology is an ancient, alternative healing practice that involves applying pressure to the hands and feet. There are specific techniques to be employed in reflexology, using just the thumb, fingers, and hands. The first known origin of reflexology traces all the way back to Egypt, as early as 2330 BC. The main principle behind the science of reflexology is that there are areas throughout the hands and feet called reflexes that correspond to each part of the body, including the glands and organs. When we use specific techniques to stimulate these reflexes, in turn we stimulate the gland, organ, or part of the body associated with the reflex, releasing energy and promoting healing in that part of the body. Reflexology is especially helpful when used as a preventative form of medicine. When performed regularly, it has been shown to help people lose weight, reduce pain caused by injuries or old age, and reduce the number of illnesses a person is prone to contracting.

Reflexology vs. Massage Therapy

It should be noted that though it may appear to be similar to massage therapy, reflexology is much different. While massage manipulates the soft tissues of the body, reflexology is focused on set and specific reflex maps, which chart the areas of the body that correspond with certain points on the hands, feet, and ears. Massage uses its own set of specific techniques to relax muscles, while the specific techniques employed in reflexology are entirely different and used to release energy in order to heal certain parts of the body.

Now that you know a little bit about this effective, all-natural, ancient type of medicine, are you ready to give it a try? Whether you believe it works for you or not, one thing is for certain: it definitely will not hurt you to try! In this book, we'll be exploring:

- How reflexology can help with weight loss
- How reflexology can eliminate stress and tension
- How to relieve pain through reflexology
- The ancient techniques of podiatry and palmistry
- How to treat illness using nature's cure

So, if you've been looking for an alternative treatment method to help you heal your body, soothe your mind, boost your mood, energy, and immune system, or help you drop some extra pounds, look no further! Dive in and explore the exciting world of reflexology and nature's cure. When you're done with this book you'll have everything you need to get started on your own healing journey using the amazing natural powers that your own body holds for you.

Chapter 1: Reflexology for Weight Loss

With obesity rates on the rise, and consequently, serious health issues like heart disease and type II diabetes becoming more prevalent and widespread, people are beginning to understand the importance of taking charge of their health. There's also mounting pressure to maintain a slim physique in a world where it seems impossible when everywhere you turn you're faced with processed, pre-made fast food that's high in fat but low on nutrients.

The weight loss battle can become terribly overwhelming for those who are constantly fighting it. Unfortunately, there is no such thing as a quick fix when it comes to losing weight long term, so you can put those weight loss pills down and cancel your packaged diet plan food. You must change your entire lifestyle, little by little, by making healthier choices in every aspect of your life, from diet to exercise and even how you think. The good news is that there are some effective and all-natural supplemental techniques and programs that can really help you drop those extra pounds, and reflexology is one of them.

Making Healthy Choices

Losing weight doesn't only effect the way you look on the outside, but how you look and feel on the inside as well. Obesity rates are at an all-time high around the world, and all of this extra weight we're carrying around can lead to some serious health complications, including heart disease, cancer, and diabetes. If you're overweight while pregnant, you and your child both run the risk of facing short-term and long-term health issues.

Don't panic! There are so many ways to begin getting your weight under control. Most importantly, don't even *think* about following one of those fad diets or fasts that all the celebrities try. When you want to lose weight, it's important to focus on making changes to your lifestyle that will last for the long-term. Many people who lose weight by following an extreme diet or fitness plan end up piling the pounds right back on as soon as their routine changes (and we all inevitably have to change our routines at one point or another).

The key to losing weight for good lies in making healthy choices. Start paying attention to your diet and start replacing some of your unhealthy options with healthier ones. Seeing a nutritionist is a very effective way to get on track with this. Additionally, you want to incorporate a little bit more exercise into your everyday life. You don't need to aspire to be a body builder, but just take the stairs every once in a while instead of the elevator and try to get a 30-minute walk in every day.

Give Reflexology a Try

Once you have decided to begin making healthier choices in your life, give reflexology a try! A healthy diet and a bit of regular physical activity supplemented with reflexology can be a very effective way to promote weight loss. Reflexology techniques for weight loss can be done at home by yourself, or if you want to be certain that you're getting the most effective results, you can see a professional reflexologist as well. A professional reflexologist can also help you by making up a diet plan to go with your reflexology sessions for weight loss.

How does it Work?

There are reflex points on your hands and feet that correspond with your digestive organs, spleen, thyroid system, and nervous system. These points should be pinpointed in order to help regulate your digestion, metabolism, and energy levels, which will help your body burn more calories and fat. When you stimulate the spleen, you will also be reducing hunger, which is a very helpful technique when trying to lose weight.

Simple Techniques for Losing Weight

If you want to try reflexology for weight loss on your own, there are some key areas of the body you'll want to focus on. The spleen, stomach and pancreas, gallbladder, and endocrine glands are all parts of your digestive system that, when stimulated, will work more efficiently and help aid in weight loss.

To get started, you'll need reflexology hand and foot charts like these:

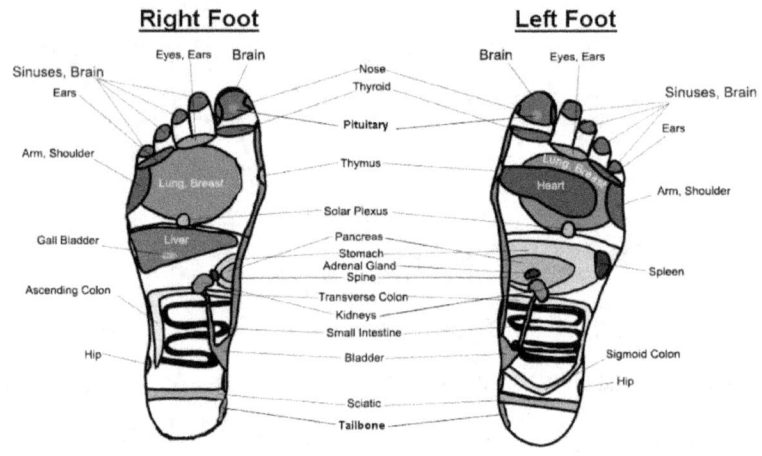

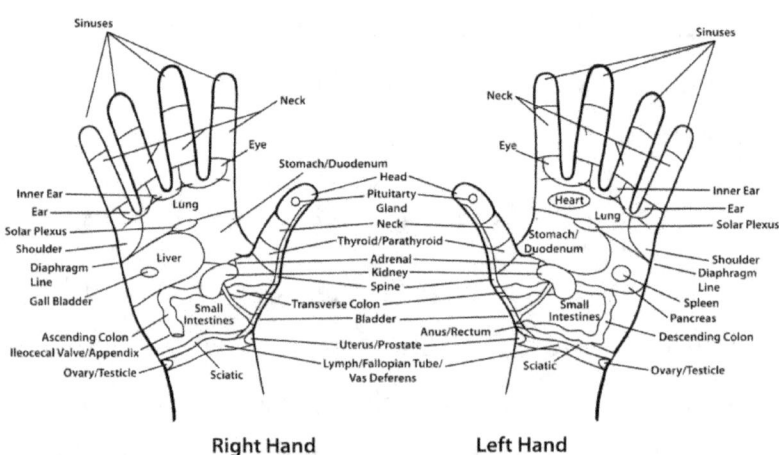

Hand Reflexology Map (palmar side)

For each exercise, find the reflex point on the foot or hand that corresponds with the part of your body you'll be working on. These exercises should be done for 5-10 minutes per day, 5 times a week and should always be performed in addition to a healthy diet and fitness routine.

Stimulate the Spleen to Reduce Hunger

Stimulate the spleen reflex by taking your left foot in your right hand and using your left thumb to work the reflex area. Do the same with the palm.

Stimulate the Stomach and Pancreas to Absorb More Nutrients

Stimulate the stomach and pancreas by taking your left foot in your right hand and pressing the corresponding reflex points using your left thumb. Move your thumb to the far limit of the reflex area and switch feet. Perform the same exercise with your palm.

Stimulate the Gallbladder to Emulsify Fat

Use the same technique as with the stomach and pancreas to work the gallbladder reflex point on the foot and palm.

Stimulate the Endocrine Glands to Regulate Hormones, Appetite, and Stress

Use your thumb and focus on applying pressure to the thyroid reflex point as well as the pituitary and adrenal glands on the foot and palm.

Chapter 2: Reflexology for Eliminating Stress and Tension

Stress: we've all experienced it before. Even the most peaceful and grounded people can feel stressed out sometimes, and that's totally okay because stress is a completely natural process. It's your body's short-term response to both bad and good experiences alike, but if you go through long-term stress, your overall well-being can take a big hit and your health can be put at risk in many different ways.

The Effects of Long-Term Stress on Your Body and Mind

If you have a stressful life full of responsibilities at home and a demanding job on top of it all, that can be very bad for your body and mind. Long-term stress might also be set off by events and situations such as physical illness, traumatic events, death, divorce, and other similar cases.

Long-term stressors such as these can have a harmful impact on your overall health and well-being, and if you don't take measures to get your stress under control, you could end up with a number of serious health issues that can ruin your quality of living and even shave precious years off your life, including:

- Depression, anxiety, irritability
- Headaches
- Insomnia
- Eating Disorders
- Substance Abuse
- Increased risk of developing

Hypertension and other issues with blood vessels
- Increased risk of stroke or heart attack
- Acid Reflux
- Stomach problems, such as nausea and/or vomiting, diarrhea or constipation
- Body Aches, especially shoulder and back pain

- In women, irregular menstrual cycles
- In men, lower levels of testosterone, leading to impotence and/or erectile dysfunction
- In men, the testes, urethra, and prostate may be more prone to infection
- Higher susceptibility to colds, flu, and other viral illnesses
- Increased risk of infection and disease
- Increased recovery time from injuries or illness

As you can see, the negative physical and mental effects of long-term stress can be very serious. But, how do we control stress when there are so many other things to worry about?

Effective Techniques for Reducing Stress and Tension

If you lead a pretty stressful life, it is imperative that you take measures to get your stress under control before it makes things even worse for you and your health. It is most important that you learn to value yourself and your quality of life enough to move your mental and physical well-being up higher on your list of everyday priorities. Often, we neglect our health until something serious happens, but you simply shouldn't do that. If you were a good friend of yours, wouldn't you have some good advice to share? Take it yourself and get a grip on your health.

There are a number of different techniques that you can practice for reducing stress. You can begin by planning a daily routine for yourself, cleaning up your diet, getting more exercise, and trying out meditation techniques at night and in the morning as well as breathing exercises throughout the day, especially when you find yourself in the middle of a stressful situation. All of these techniques will help give you a greater sense of calm, control, and inner peace.

Employ Reflexology Techniques for Effective Stress Relief

There are specific reflex points on your hands, forearms, and feet that reduce stress when you press and knead them. Massaging these reflex points for just one minute is especially effective when combined with breathing exercises to reduce stress and tension. You can easily massage these points on your own anytime you're feeling stressed out or at night before sleeping.

Use the forearm point to regulate your heart rate, relax your body and mind, and stimulate circulation

The forearm point is located at your wrist, between the tendons that run up the inside of your forearm. To find the sweet spot, simply measure the width of your thumb times two, up the middle of your forearm from the crease between your hand and wrist.

Press the reflex point here, between the tendons, and knead it, using short circular movements. You'll feel a small amount of comfortable pain when you're doing it properly.

Working this reflex point also helps relieve and treat heart palpitations, insomnia, nausea, and vomiting.

Use the wrist point to calm your mind and relax your body

There is a reflex point located on either side of your wrist, on the crease between the wrist and forearm that is effective at calming the mind and relaxing the body when you work it properly. Press the point at the end of your wrist, just inside the wrist bone end. Knead this reflex point using the same motions you used on your forearm.

Working this reflex point also helps relieve heart palpitations, insomnia, emotional upsets, and memory issues.

Use the foot point to relax, relieve anxiety, and get better sleep

If you refer to the foot chart in chapter one, you can see the point on the bottom of the foot at the bottom of the areas connected with the lungs and breast. Press that point, in the middle of your foot, hard enough to feel a slight, comfortable pain. Hold the point for one or two minutes and repeat on the other foot.

Additionally, you may refer to the hand and foot charts in chapter one of this book, and focus on working the reflex points for the kidneys, spleen, heart, and liver. These organs are deeply connected with anxiety and emotional stress, so it is recommended to work on them if you wish to release energy in these areas.

Chapter 3: Reflexology for Pain Relief

When you get sick, stressed out, or experience an injury, your muscles tense up and cause a lot of tension-induced pain throughout the body. You know, those random neck and back aches and sharp pains that never seem to cease no matter how much you rub and massage the area? When rubbing and kneading these sore spots isn't doing the trick and medication just isn't enough, there are fortunately some very effective natural treatments and techniques that will help you ease the pain.

Ease Your Pain Using Effective Reflexology Techniques

Reflexology techniques are very effective on easing pain in the back, head, shoulders, and neck that has been caused by exhaustion, stress, or mild physical injuries. It works by applying pressure, kneading, or massaging the reflex points on the hands and feet that correspond with the spine, neck and shoulder areas, and shoulder areas.

When done properly, these techniques are extremely effective at easing mild aches and pains. It should be noted, however, that they will probably not be effective for relieving serious pain caused by serious injuries, or on long term, extreme pain. In these cases, speak to your doctor about supplementing reflexology treatment with your standard treatments. At least it will help relieve stress, which is sure to take some aches and pains away!

Reflexology for Mild Back Pain

When you've been on your feet all day, made it through an intense workout, or are just plain exhausted, reflexology techniques can help seriously ease your back pain.

Use the foot chart in chapter one to locate the reflex point for the spine area on the inside of your foot. Use the palms of your hands to hold your foot, keeping your thumbs on the bottom and fingers on the top. Then, gently and slowly twist your hands in opposite directions. Perform this exercise for just 30 seconds to relax.

When you're done with the relaxation technique, use your thumb to "walk" up the spine reflex point. Start at the bottom of the heel and walk your thumb up to the tip of your big toe. Repeat from the tow down to the heel. Next, perform this technique, but instead of walking horizontal, press in a vertical motion, moving down the length of the inside of your foot.

Go through the thumb walks twice, and finish the exercise with the relaxation technique you began with. Perform the exercise on the other foot.

Reflexology for Shoulder and Mild Neck Pain

When your shoulders start aching after a long day, or you feel stabbing pain while you're working, perform this reflexology technique to help ease the pain.

Begin by performing the horizontal thumb walk technique that we reviewed for mild back pain. Start with the right foot.

When you're done with the thumb walk, use the chart in chapter one to locate the reflex point on the foot that is connected with the neck and perform the thumb walk across this reflex point, moving up, down, and diagonal. Go over this spot 1-2 times.

Then, locate the reflex point that corresponds with the shoulders and perform the thumb walk in the same way you did it for the neck point. Repeat this over the top of the foot in the same reflex point for the shoulders. Then, gently massage the notch of the bone under your small toe on the outer edge of the foot. Do this for about 30 seconds.

When you're done with all of these exercises on the right foot, repeat the same on the left foot.

Reflexology for Headaches

Headaches are painful and uncomfortable and they can be very distracting and annoying. If you experience a headache and need some fast relief, try a simple reflexology technique.

First, place the palm of one hand on your stomach for support. Then, use your thumb and index finger to gently hold the base joint of your thumb, where the thumb connects to your hand. Massage the area by rolling the joint in one direction for a full circle, then move the same way in the opposite direction.

Next, move your fingers up and hold the reflex point just above the second thumb joint. Then, twist in a gentle side-to-side motion for five seconds, and use a circular motion to rotate in one direction for five seconds, and then switch directions for another five seconds. Do this for each joint on every finger on the hand.

Lastly, use all of the fingers and the thumb on your massaging hand and squeeze the thumb, moving up and down and around all sides. Do this for each finger on the hand.

Switch hands and repeat these techniques for the other hand.

Chapter 4: Treating Illness using Nature's Cures

There have been some exciting advancements in the medical industry over the last few decades, but that doesn't mean that all is perfect in the world of modern medicine. Despite the advancements, many people have become distrustful towards modern doctors and practitioners, and are beginning to seek out natural and holistic cures for a myriad of illnesses and diseases.

Look to Nature to Find a Cure

The problem with many modern treatments that include prescription medication for patients today is that they do not get to the root of a person's health issues to completely solve them, but instead, in many cases, the medication relieves some symptoms of the illness or disease while new issues arise from the side effects of the medication. So the patient then has to take a new medication to combat those side effects, and that's how the cycle begins. Some people with diabetes, cancer, and other diseases are on dozens of medications when some of these people could actually find cures through nature if they were to take a holistic route to healing instead of following modern medicine.

It is not so much a common practice for a modern practitioner to ask a patient about their diet and lifestyle when they come to them with an ailment, but these are the first areas where one should investigate. A poor diet and lifestyle is sometimes where any given illness begins, and likewise is usually where one can be most effectively treated.

Reflexology: A Supplemental Treatment Method

In order to effectively treat any given illness or disease using nature's cures, one must combine a variety of techniques and treatment methods to create an overall well-balanced diet and lifestyle. There is no specific holistic method that will cure any ailment on its own, but when you combine the proper diet, exercise, and supplemental treatment methods for your specific ailment and body type, you've got the recipe for a winning cure that is likely to be more effective than any modern medication on the market.

There are foods and herbs that work to heal certain parts of the body and get rid of illness, and likewise there are certain foods and herbs that should be avoided depending on what you're afflicted with. Specific exercises and holistic treatments can work to relieve symptoms, clear blocked energy, and promote detoxification within the body, which is extremely effective for treating a wide range of illnesses and diseases.

How Can Reflexology Help?

Reflexology is an ancient practice that has been used throughout centuries to promote healing within the body by clearing blocked energy, promoting detoxification, and restoring the natural equilibrium within the body. It is most effective as a supplemental treatment to relieve pain and help the body heal itself.

Reflexology is especially effective in bringing relief from symptoms that arise from the following ailments, illnesses, and diseases:

- Respiratory issues and breathing disorders
- Sinus issues
- Bowel and other digestive disorders caused by stress
- Irregularities and imbalances of hormones
- Trouble sleeping
- Post-op recovery
- Musculoskeletal pain, especially in the back, neck, and shoulders
- Nausea induced by chemotherapy or other harsh medical treatments
- Fibromyalgia

Although reflexology has not been accepted into standard modern medicine yet, doctors and scientists are working to validate this ancient practice and introduce it into modern medicine as a valid form of therapy. So far, clinical studies have been able to identify a number of major health benefits related to reflexology, including:

- Positive balance and maintenance of blood pressure and immune system
- Positive respiratory function
- Pain relief from musculoskeletal problems and during post-op recovery
- Balance in blood sugar levels
- Bowel function improvements
- Lowering levels of anxiety and stress
- PMS relief and lower labor times in women
- Relief from sinus problems, headaches, and migraines

So, whether you're suffering from asthma, diabetes, allergies, anxiety, back, neck, or shoulder pain, PMS, digestive problems, headaches, or migraines, reflexology as a supplemental treatment method will surely help balance your body and mind to provide you with some much-needed relief.

Reflexology Techniques for Illness

For the most effective relief and treatment for post-op pain and issues caused by serious injury or disease, you should see a professional reflexologist at least four times per week. These experts will perform the ancient techniques that they are well versed in and will be able to customize a treatment plan for you, including diet and nutrition tips, which will seriously help aid in your recovery.

There are, however, some simple techniques that you can try on yourself anytime that will help to relieve sinus pressure, swollen glands, nausea and vomiting, and sore throat. These are the most common inflictions normally caused by allergies, the common cold, and flu. Reflexology is especially effective in providing relief from these symptoms.

Relieve a Sore Throat Using Reflex Points on the Hands

There are many bones and joints in the fingers and toes that correspond with the top of the neck and the bones in the skull and jaw, which is the area you want to focus on when you're suffering from a sore throat. This reflexology technique is similar to the headache technique shared in chapter three.

First, place the palm of one hand on your stomach for support. Then, use your thumb and index finger to gently hold the base joint of your thumb, where the thumb connects to your hand. Massage the area by rolling the joint in one direction for a full circle, then move the same way in the opposite direction.

Next, move your fingers up and hold the reflex point just above the second thumb joint. Then, twist in a gentle side-to-side motion for five seconds, and use a circular motion to rotate in one direction for five seconds, and then switch directions for another five seconds. Do this for each joint on every finger on the hand.

Lastly, use all of the fingers and the thumb on your massaging hand and squeeze the thumb, moving up and down and around all sides. Do this for each finger on the hand.

Switch hands and repeat these techniques for the other hand.

Cool the Wrists to Relieve Nausea and Vomiting

The wrists are essential reflex points because they connect all of the energy meridians located on the hands to the rest of the body. So, when these points are cooled, it cools the entire body, immediately relieving nausea.

Use cold running water or something cold like ice, frozen vegetables, a cold piece of metal, a cold wall, or something similar. Run the water over the insides of your wrists, where the lines are between the hand and the arm, with your palms facing up. If you don't have water, place something cold on your wrists at the same point or hold them against something cold. Do this for 30 seconds to 2 minutes, or however long it takes for your nausea to subside.

Work the Toes to Relieve Swollen Glands

When you experience mild swelling in the glands, you want to focus on working the gland point reflexes on the feet. The technique to relieve headaches, shared in chapter three, is also effective when used in addition to the gland point techniques.

Begin by rotating the big toe on your right foot by holding it at the base and moving it gently back and forth in circular motions. The purpose is to stretch and rotate this base joint. Move up the toe and work the same motion for the top joint. Gently repeat this exercise for each toe.

After you rotate the smallest toe, perform a thumb walk over your toes, starting with the big toe. You do this by pressing your thumb horizontally over the base of the toes. Use the chart in chapter one to locate the reflex point areas for the thyroid and pituitary glands and perform a gentle thumb walk across these regions, moving in an upward motion across, diagonal, and down. Perform this technique for one minute.

Clear Blocked Sinuses by Pressing the Tips of Your Fingers and Toes

The tips of your fingers and toes are connected with your sinuses, which can become blocked for a number of reasons. This is always a very uncomfortable situation that can make it difficult for you to focus or think. If you need some fast relief from sinus blockage, try this simple reflexology technique to increase the blood circulation through your sinuses and help you breathe again.

Use the charts in chapter one to locate the reflex points for the sinus area, at the tips of your fingers and toes. Begin with the thumb of your right hand and squeeze the sides of the tip in a pulsating movement for five seconds, then repeat this movement in the center of the tip, at the topmost point of the thumb. Move to the index finger and repeat the same movement. Do this for each finger and then switch hands.

The same technique should be applied to the reflex points for the sinuses located on the toes.

Conclusion: Use Ancient Techniques for Optimal Health

It is important to understand that ancient techniques like reflexology are not meant to work as substitutes for another treatment method, but are extremely helpful when used as a supplement to a treatment method.

When ancient techniques are combined and applied properly, they positively have the potential to lead a person to optimal health, because they follow the cures that nature has laid out for all of us.

The Problem with Quick Fixes

There's a big problem in the world today with industries straying further and further from nature, pushing us to live in ways that nature did not intend for us to live. Many people contract illnesses and disease as a result of toxins building up in the body due to poor environment combined with an improper diet and poor lifestyle choices. It's all too common today for us to seek out quick fixes, whether they be through food or medicine, we don't have the time to wait for anything.

Many people today have been made to believe that they just don't have the time, money, or resources to live a natural, healthy lifestyle. The world and the people in it are being thrown off balance, and it is now more important than ever before to ensure that we don't lose sight of important ancient techniques and nature's cures.

One reason why many people may be quick to dismiss the ancient and natural route to healing is because it is not usually a quick fix. In order to employ nature's cures and ancient healing techniques in the ways we need to in order to see the positive results and feel the healing effects, we must be willing to undergo some serious lifestyle changes. It takes a bit of time and a bit of patience, but if you begin these practices as preventative measures, you may never even be faced with the challenge of finding a cure for a disease that would have inflicted you due to negligence of nature's ways.

Your Body Can Heal Itself

The beautiful thing about reflexology and all other holistic treatments, ancient healing techniques, and natural cures is that they're usually simply prompting the body to heal itself. Our bodies are amazing, magnificent, and miraculous things that are capable of working wonders – and *do* work wonders – every moment of every day. When we lose sight of the miraculous ways our bodies are able to function, blocking our energy and preventing our systems from running at their optimal capabilities, we need to get back on to nature's path and find the cures laid out for us through ancient times.

Unblock Your Energy

Many natural cures and ancient healing techniques deal with unblocking the energy in the body, allowing the natural processes to flow better, thus promoting better function of every organ and system throughout the body.

Lower Your Stress

We must understand the importance of maintaining low stress levels as well. As we discussed earlier, long-term stress can lead to a number of serious health complications, and at the very least it can make a person uncomfortable by causing a lot of aches and pains throughout the body. Ancient healing techniques often deal with eliminating stress as it is the root cause of the onset of many illnesses and diseases.

Maintain a Balanced Diet and Lifestyle

Another cause for the onset of many illnesses and diseases is maintaining a poor diet and lifestyle, which is another area that most ancient techniques and natural cures really focus on. Our bodies were not meant to be stuffed full of synthetic foods, chemicals, and toxins. When we eat processed foods, meats injected with antibiotics and hormones, drink alcohol and sugary drinks, or worse yet, drinks packed with cancer-causing sugar substitutes, we are prohibiting our bodies to function at their optimum potential. In addition to following reflexology techniques, it is imperative to eat healthy, natural foods and live an active lifestyle to allow our bodies the equilibrium they need to function optimally and heal themselves.

Get to the Root of the Issue

The purpose of these ancient healing techniques and natural cures is not to provide another quick fix with a chemical cure, but to get to the root of the issue. These techniques and cures are very much focused on the individual, and are rarely, if ever, designed and available as a cure-all for everyone. Each of us lives a different life and may be afflicted by similar ailments for completely different reasons. Holistic treatment methods focus on getting to the root of the problem and finding out where it began and everything that has contributed to its growth, in order to work on balancing the systems of the body back out, allowing it to grow strong enough to heal itself as it should be able to.

Supplement Your Routine with Reflexology

You don't need to be suffering from an injury, illness, or disease to try the reflexology techniques outlined in this book. It's great to use reflexology as a supplemental preventative treatment in conjunction with a balanced diet and an active lifestyle.

If you are suffering from an injury, illness, or disease and would like to use reflexology as a supplement to your existing treatment method, it would be best to get in touch with a reflexology specialist who can suggest a great course of treatment for you.

No matter how you decide to use the effective ancient techniques of reflexology, always make sure you combine them with a natural and healthy diet, a reasonable amount of exercise, and a low-stress lifestyle for the best results. There's a cure for everything hidden in nature. It's up to us to discover the benefits!

References

http://www.takingcharge.csh.umn.edu/explore-healing-practices/reflexology

http://www.reflexology-usa.net/facts.htm

http://www.how-to-do-reflexology.com/reflexologyforweightloss.html

http://reflexology-map.com/reflexology-for-weight-loss/

http://www.healthline.com/health/stress/effects-on-body

http://www.chinese-holistic-health-exercises.com/reflexology-for-anxiety.html

http://www.how-to-do-reflexology.com/reflexologyfor.html

http://www.energybenefits.com/phdi/p1.nsf/supppages/6657?opendocument&part=2

www.ingramcontent.com/pod-product-compliance
Lightning Source LLC
Chambersburg PA
CBHW070842310526
45793CB00011B/502